How To

Return

Beauty
and
Clear Vision

Back to Your Eyes

A Practical Course for Anyone with Poor Eyesight
By Jane Kabarguina

Copyright © Jane Kabarguina 2008

The Certificate of Registration of Copyright is issued pursuant to sections 49 and 53 of the Canadian Copyright Act.

Email: info@snezha.com
Website: www.snezha.com

All rights reserved.
No part of this book may be reproduced or used
in any form or by any means, electronic or mechanical,
without prior permission in writing from the Author.

Initial front cover design, and text pictures by Jane Kabarguina
Editing and book formatting by Patricia McSmith
Photography by Jane Kabarguina and Andre Beskorsy

> This book does not represent, in any way, orthodox medical opinion. The findings herein presented are all natural methods as passed down from the wisest and most knowledgeable men and women throughout the methods cited herein may do for an individual in any given case. The author and publishers assume no obligation or liability as to how any one may use or misuse this information. Those with eye injuries, eye disease, and/or degenerative eye conditions consult with a professional eye specialist or physician.

CONTENTS

- CONTENTS 3
- Part 1 5
  - Chapter 1 – Introduction 5
  - Chapter 2 – My Personal Journey 5
- Part 2 8
  - Chapter 1 – Eye Relaxation Exercises ... 8
  - Chapter 2 – Fixation and Stretching 9
  - Chapter 3 – Rolling Movements 21
  - Chapter 4 – Palming 23
  - Chapter 5 – Acupressure 27
  - Chapter 6 – Dynamic Set 36
  - Chapter 8 – Focusing Exercises 46
  - Chapter 9 – Watching the Sun 50
  - Chapter 10 – Observations from My Experience 52
- Part 3 57
  - Chapter 1 – Nutrition 58
  - Chapter 2 – Recipes 59
  - Chapter 3 – Herbal Medicine 62
- Part 4 63
  - Chapter 1 – Posture and Spine Exercises 63
  - Chapter 2 – Eye Beauty 69
  - Chapter 3 – Natural Eyelid Lifting 71

References – **74**

Part 1

Chapter 1 - Introduction

Yes, it is that simple! Just by exercising certain parts of your body, your muscles become firm, fit, healthy and good looking. The same happens with your eyes - by exercising your eyes, muscles that hold the eyeballs in place are strengthened, blood circulation around the eye improves, skin around the eyes become toned, eyebrow twitching disappears, sensitivity to light, wind and dryness fades away, perfect vision comes back, and your eyes shine like they did in youth! You might consider these as positive side effects from what is called "Eye Exercising".

Chapter 2 – My Personal Journey

I have been wearing glasses since I was in Grade 4. It began due to the fact that I was not able to see anything written on the chalkboard from sitting in the fifth row in the class. I complained that I could not concentrate when sitting that far back, and then I was transferred to the first row. When I found out that I couldn't see from the first row, the teacher complained to my Grandma that I am squinting my eyes and not able to copy down the required homework from the chalkboard.

Well, my Grandma and I ended up at the doctor's office, and naturally, they prescribed eyeglasses for me. But the problem was that the deterioration of my vision continued and I had to change prescriptions twice, going to a lower number of diopters and thicker lenses each time.

I was always very embarrassed wearing glasses. When I was studying at the University in Siberia, I was one of the first patients that tried hand-crafted glass lenses. It was such an inconvenience to take care of them – washing them everyday in the soap solution, boiling them every week, de-sanitizing them every month and the constant fear of losing them.

Then Bausch & Lomb came out with their soft, revolutionary contact lenses. But the problem with their soft lenses arises from the fact that they always have to be wet. In order to keep up with the humidity level, these lenses suck moisture from the eyes and people, like myself, simply get migraine headaches from the eyes constantly being dried out.

Time passed. I was wearing thick-lense glasses again. Then I decided to do some research on hard lenses. There was still a certain level of inconvenience associated with them. For example, if it's windy, or your eye lashes are too long and they curl into your eyes and you blink from time to time, or if you are wearing mascara, or if you are in sports, you are completely inconvenienced with the hard lenses! You will be either in pain or on your knees looking to see where these expensive lenses went.

I then decided to go back to glasses – super light-weight designer framed, extra-thin lenses with anti-glare coating. There has been tremendous improvement in the glasses-making technology in the past decade. But glasses are still glasses - they are not part of your beautiful body and the fact that you are wearing them already indicates that something is not balanced or working perfectly in your mind and/or body. And it doesn't matter how fancy and pretty your glasses are – you are still wearing glasses!

Finally, I ended up contemplating laser surgery. After researching the eye surgery clinics, prices, locations, websites, radio commercials, friend's experiences etc., I walked into one of the clinics in Toronto (Canada) to learn everything I could about their procedures and results. I was given a thick brochure to read before I was called for an eye examination. When I read through the brochure's material, I was left in emotional shock – more than half of the material was talking about complications that may occur during or after the laser surgery procedure. The complication percentage is very little – just 4%! But I do not want to be part of the 4% under any circumstances! And the surgery is performed on both of the eyes almost simultaneously. If something goes wrong, then both of your eyes are left blind.

I decided that this is not an option for me. What else could I do?

I remembered that I stopped my vision failure in fourth grade by doing eye exercises. Apparently, there has been plenty of literature written about improving your eyesight naturally in many languages, which already proves that it **is** possible. Luckily, I was able to do my research in two languages – English and Russian, which allowed me to be introduced to a few different schools including European, Chinese, Indian, Russian, Korean, Japanese, and others.

I tried all of them.

All of them worked. But during my experience with all of the different techniques I tried while researching, I discovered a flexible system that combines all of the different schools together, taking the best parts of each of them and at the same time, not exhausting the person that is beginning to step on their path to vision improvement.

What follows are the results that came out of the research that made my eyes healthy again.

Part 2

Chapter 1 – Eye Relaxation Exercises

Most of the eye exercising routines that are already published do not include eye relaxation techniques or, if they do include them, they don't pay enough attention or spend enough time doing them. But I have found that this is the most important procedure.

And the result of not including eye relaxation techniques are either you get pain in your eye sockets and give up exercising your eyes, or you search for the eye improvement instructor. In order to prevent this situation, I am introducing relaxing tips and tricks before the main part of the eye exercises. This book is organized in such a specific way that it will always push you to perform eye relaxation exercises no matter what stage you are at. The relaxation part of your eye exercises is placed right at the beginning of this practical course, stressing the fact that before exercising any part of your body, you must relax the muscles first and ensure that they are in the best condition and ready for any type of training. There are also multiple types of eye relaxation tricks throughout the different levels of the eye exercises.

Relaxation Exercise #1

Close your eyes halfway down. You will notice that your upper eyelids constantly tremble with different amplitude. Concentrate your efforts on stopping this trembling. Little hint – it will be easier to achieve if you look at objects further away.

Relaxation Exercise #2

Slowly close your eyes, like your eyelids are made of puffy, cottony clouds. Now feel that your eyes are getting extremely comfortable in this position. Imagine the place behind the eyes getting warm and feel the blood, filled with oxygen, flowing through your eye sockets. When you inhale, imagine the breezy oxygenized air coming through your nose into your eyes, washing each eye's blood vessel. Exhale through your mouth. Breathe this way for one or two minutes and end this exercise with a smile.

Relaxation Exercise #3

Imagine two dots on a wall, one being half a meter from the other one. Slowly look at one dot, then move your gaze to the other dot, then slowly look back to the first dot. Continue doing these movements while imagining that you are a lazy cat who is falling asleep, but still keep your attention to the fly on the wall. Soon your eyes will feel that they
are heavy …
very heavy …
they begin to feel like they are made out of steel …

Chapter 2 – Fixation and Stretching

Wake up! It is morning!

Begin the day with lightly massaging your bottom eyelids in a circular motion using your middle fingers.

Then blink for a half a minute. Try to do that with adequate speed, and at the same time, make the movements very light. Imagine that your eyelashes are butterfly's wings. The process of blinking is extremely important to your eyes – it relaxes most of the eye muscles and lubricates and cleanses the eyeballs. Little hint – if you are not satisfied with the speed of your blinking, try to smile at the same time – the speed will immediately increase!

Now draw an imaginary horizontal line between your eyebrows (a mirror and marker can really help your imagination), then draw a vertical line up from your nose. If you are good at geometry, you will be able to find the point where these two lines cross each other. This point of intersection will be slightly above the bridge of your nose. Then you have to fix your gaze on this spot (this is the most difficult part) and most importantly, try to keep your gaze in this position for a few seconds. Your eyes will start closing down by themselves. Return your gaze back to straight ahead and close your eyes to relax them. Some people can even meditate in this position.

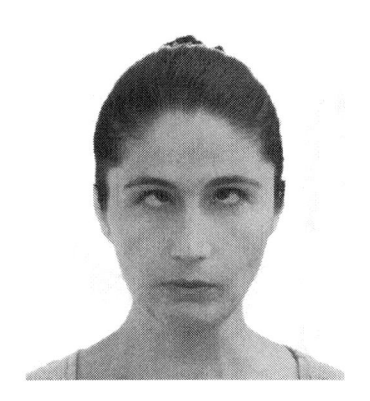

If you wish to continue even after this relaxing procedure, you will need to concentrate your vision on another important spot – the tip of your nose (in yoga practice it is called NASAGRA-DRASHTY). Keep your gaze in this position for a short time (everyone is different, evaluate how long is best for you) and then return your gaze to straight ahead. Close your eyes. These two concentrative staring procedures are considered to be deep relaxation for a few eye muscles.

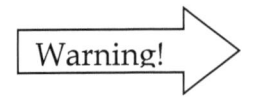

Warning! → What happens if you don't do ANY relaxing techniques before, between and after eye exercises?

Let's imagine for a second that you decided to do a split like an Olympic gymnast. What is going to happen if you have never tried to stretch your legs before that decision? The answer is very simple - if you are not a little child, you will simply tear the ligaments that connect your legs to your body and you will be in pain for at least two to three months.

In the case of eye exercising, you may get pain or a clicking noise in your eye sockets, ache in the sinuses or even a major headache. Therefore, it is strongly recommended that you do eye relaxing exercises before, after and many times during different types of eye exercises. I also recommend performing any kind of relaxation techniques whenever you feel that your eyes are tired (such as when working at the computer, watching a movie, sewing, knitting, etc.).

Warming Up

Sit (or stand) straight, make sure that your shoulder blades touch the chair's back (or wall if you are standing), chin up, stomach in, chest out and shoulders down. Now you are ready to begin.

1. Hold your head straight and look to your extreme left side and try to keep your eyes in that position.

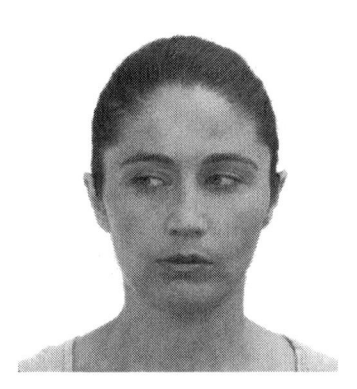

Return your gaze and look straight in front of you. Blink for a few seconds. Repeat 2 - 3 times. Then relax your eyes with blinking.

2. Hold your head straight and look to your extreme right side and try to keep your eyes in this position (try to do this for the same length of time as the left eye). Return your gaze and look straight in front of you.

Blink for a few seconds. Repeat 2 - 3 times. Then relax your eyes with blinking.

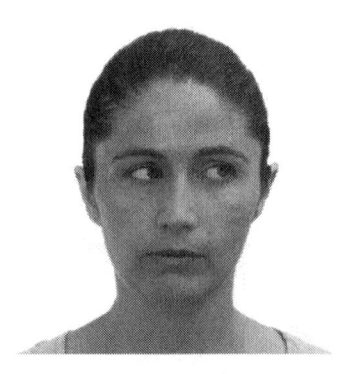

3. Look up and hold, then return the gaze back. Blink for a few seconds. Repeat 2 - 3 times. Relax your eyes with blinking.

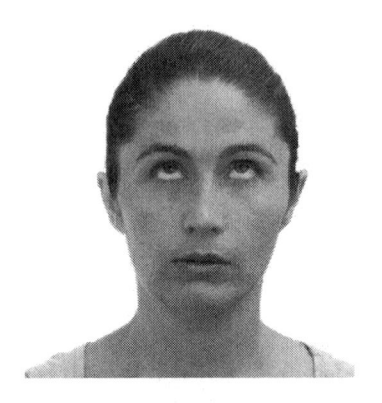

4. Look down and hold, then return the gaze back. Blink for a few seconds. Repeat 2 - 3 times. Relax your eyes with blinking.

    Realize that it is called "Eye Exercises" because you only need to move your eyes, not your head!

5. Now return your head to the original position (remember to keep your posture straight). Look at the right top corner and hold your gaze there. Then return it back. Blink for a few seconds. Repeat 2 - 3 times. Relax your eyes with blinking.

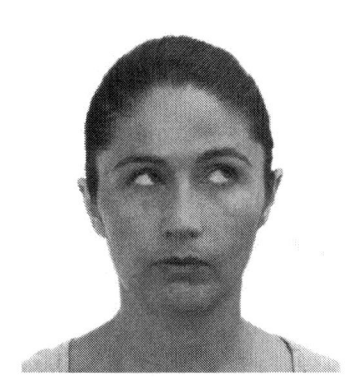

6. The next position for the eyes is the right bottom corner. This is a little bit more complicated. Let's look at your right shoulder - that is exactly the right bottom corner for your gaze (if you are still keeping your posture). Fix your eyes in that direction without moving your head.

   Hold your eyesight in that pose for a period of time, and then look straight ahead again. Repeat 2 - 3 times and relax your eyes with blinking.

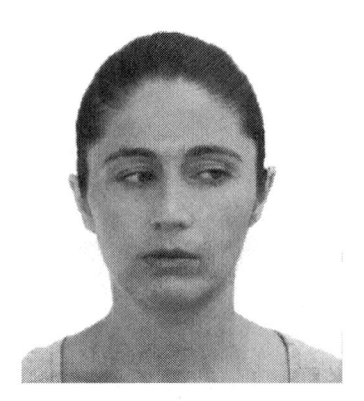

7. While still trying to keep your head straight, look down to the bottom left – at your left shoulder. Try to fixate the eye position there, and then look straight ahead again. Repeat 2 -3 times and relax your eyes with blinking.

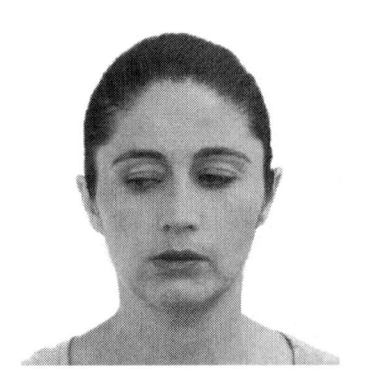

8. And the only corner remaining is the upper left one, somewhere above your left temple. Try to concentrate and fixate the eye position there. Then look straight ahead again. Repeat 2 – 3 times and relax your eyes with blinking.

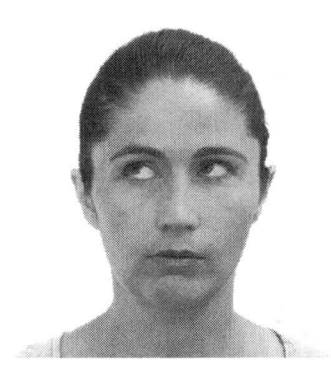

Let's end the stretching exercises with some fun stuff! Look around and find one object that is small enough and pretend that it is a black dot.

Start staring at that dot and at the same time turn your head to the right side as much as you can while keeping your eyes fixed on that dot.

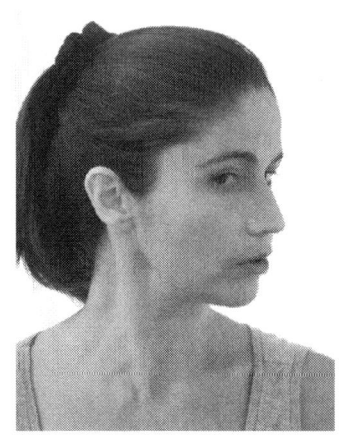

Now slowly move your head to the left side, still keeping your eyes staring at the same dot.

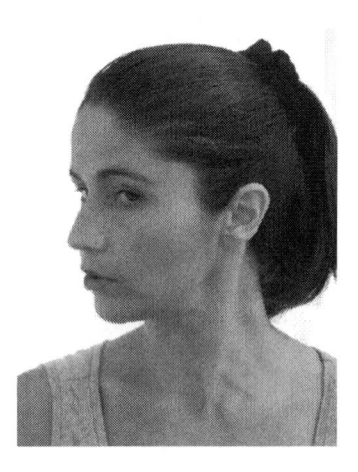

I usually suggest performing eye exercises when you are alone, or, at least, when nobody sees your eyes because you can look very funny!

Now blink for a few seconds and continue the fun by lifting your nose up (and therefore, your head also), keeping your eyes on the same dot.

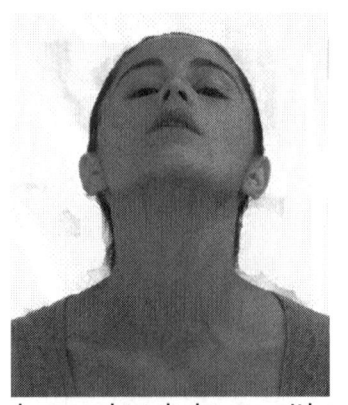

Now bend your head down without taking your eyes off the dot. Experiment with different head positions, always keeping your gaze still on the same dot.

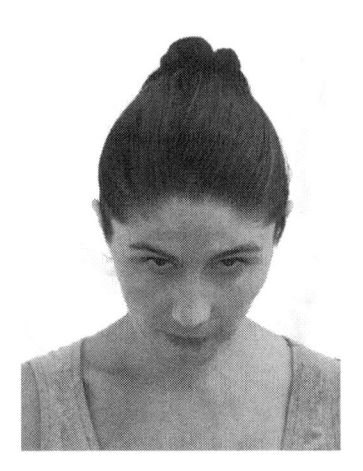

Finish up by rolling circles with your head, keeping your eyes on the same dot. There are no strict rules about this exercise – you can simply move your head in any direction you want to, just keep your gaze on the same dot.

Now let's relax your eyes with different type of blinking – shut your eyes really tight, even tighter, and then open them as wide as you can.

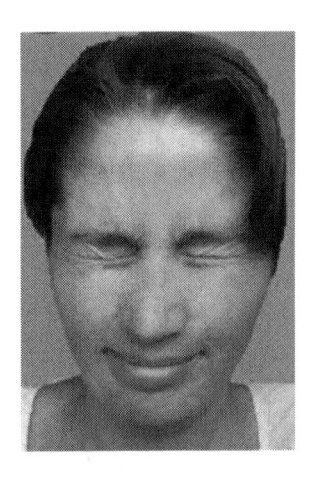

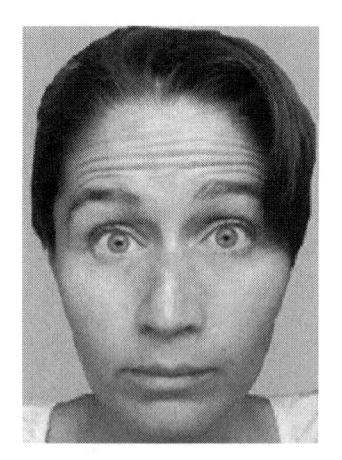

Tears may burst out of your eyes at that moment. This is exactly what we want to achieve – getting the tears out will lubricate your eyes!

Repeat this exercise a few times. I suggest you do this kind of eye relaxation procedure whenever you feel that your eyes are tired, such as in front of the computer, while reading a book, standing in a lineup at the store, and especially during commercials while you are watching TV. You will look at commercials from a different perspective – use that time for yourself! Execute eye relaxation procedures, floss your teeth, work on abdominals, stretch your spine, jump rope or stand on your head, all in front of the television.

Chapter 3 – Rolling Movements

Now that your eye muscles are warmed up, you are ready for something more complicated – Eye Math. Do not get scared - all you need to know is what the number eight looks like.

Let's draw this number eight with your eyes, in a clockwise direction, imagining that this number eight is lying on its side horizontally:

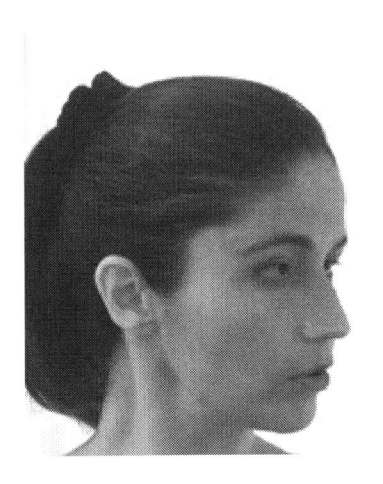

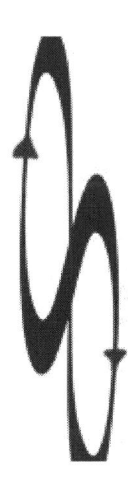

Try to move your eyes very slowly without cutting any edges. Mathematicians even came up with a name for the horizontal eight - they call it **infinity**.

When you draw about seven of these "number eights", change the direction of drawing to a counter clockwise direction and repeat the drawing. Follow up with blinking to relax the eyes.

After that, go ahead with drawing a vertical "number eight" with your eyes (seven times in a clockwise direction and seven times in a counter-clockwise direction). Follow up with blinking.

Now close your eyes and repeat this entire math drawing of "figure eights" ∞ and **8** with your eyes closed. Even the blinking part has to be done with closed eyes. By the way, blinking with closed eyes is also considered a relaxation technique. It is also a very good exercise for your eyelids, especially the upper ones. Do not forget about your breathing. Don't slow it down and, most importantly, during the entire eye exercising procedures, try to remember to breathe calmly and deeply.

The next exercise requires a high level of concentration. Make sure that you keep your posture straight (chest out, stomach in, etc.). Look up and start drawing a circle with your eyes in a clockwise direction. Try to make the circle as perfect as possible without cutting any angles. Complete 7 - 8 rounds, and then blink for a minute.

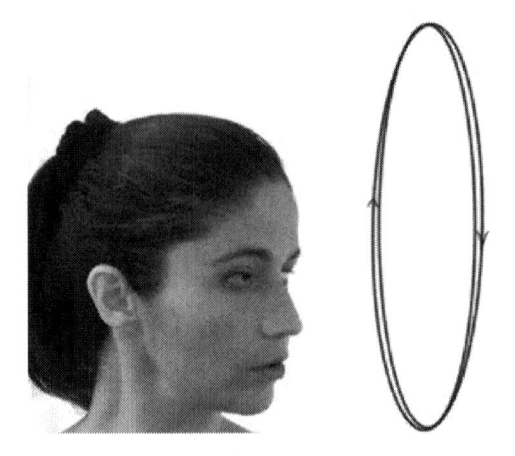

When completed, change the direction to counter-clockwise and draw another set of circles. You may notice that your eyes may hurt a little when they are going through a certain angle of the circle. Then repeat the circular movements in both directions again, but with your eyes closed.

Even if you had any stresses or thoughts that would not leave your mind before you started to do an eye stretching set or rolling eye movements, they should disappear by now. You are maintaining a very high level of concentration.

Do not open your eyes. Keep them closed, concentrating all your attention on the eye sockets. Feel the warmth behind your eyes. Now relax your bottom eye eyelids, upper eyelids, and eyebrows.

Spread the relaxation to your forehead, your mouth, lips, ears, and the back of your head. Finally, bring the relaxation up to the crown of your head. Stay in this position for a short time.

Actually, now is the perfect time to introduce you to one of the most powerful eye relaxation techniques that we all perform unconsciously when our eyes are tired.

Chapter 4 - Palming

Palming means covering closed eyes with your palms. There are a few ways to perform palming - you just need to choose the method you feel the most comfortable with.

Method 1 - Used to be My Favorite

Remember when you played hide and seek as a child? You covered your eyes with your palms and you weren't supposed to see anybody! Just do the same thing you did in your childhood - cup your eyes with your palms and observe the darkness in front of your face. Make sure you are not touching your eyelids with your palms.

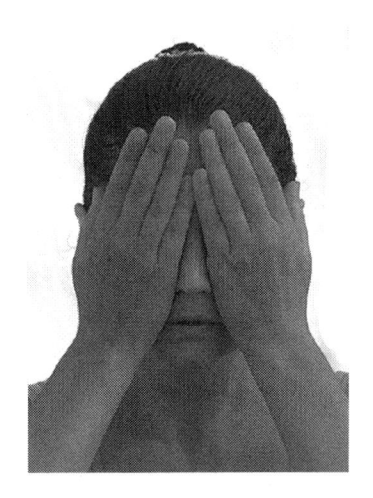

Method 2 - Yoga Method

Warm up your hands - rub the palms against each other or hold them under hot water (not too hot!). Prepare your palms like on the picture.

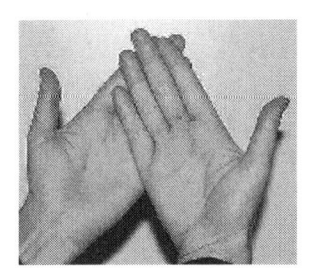

The base of your right pinkie will be on the base of your left pinkie, or if it is more comfortable, place your left palm on top of the right palm, making an upside down letter "V" with your palms.

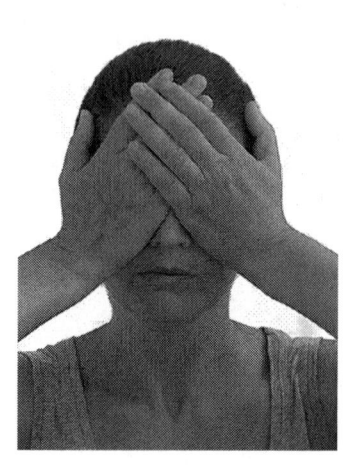

Look at the palms with your eyes. The base of the pinkie fingers will be right on the bridge of your nose. Make sure you are able to breathe through your nose, otherwise adjust the location of your palms and fingers. Next, leaving your eyes open, turn towards the light (sun, light fixtures, etc.) and check out the position of your palms.

If you are able to see the light through any of the holes between your fingers, correct the placement of your palms until you get perfect cover that does not allow any light to your eyes. Now you are ready for the deepest eye relaxation technique that also relaxes and calms your whole neurological system. Do not concentrate on the eyes or area behind them.

Breathe deeply. Focus just on your breathing (it helps to fully relax). Just concentrate on how you inhale, exhale, inhale, exhale…

Feel the warmth coming from your palms. Then imagine absolutely black space in front of your eyes. I found that in the beginning, it could be an extremely difficult task to perform. The worse your vision is, the more difficult it is to picture absolutely black space. But I was able to trick my mind. I recalled drawing different shapes with the black pencil. For example, I would picture in my mind how I draw a circle and then how I would shade it in with the same black pencil. Just go ahead – find what tricks work for your mind. I have also tried picturing a starry sky and I was removing stars one by one with black clouds.

This method is perfect for the relaxation of the whole mind and body. Sometimes it takes a few minutes to get the relaxation level needed, but other times it is almost immediate. It doesn't matter that you might not succeed in the beginning, just continue trying and remember – whoever looks will find!

There is also another important point that needs to be taken into consideration – the head and neck position. Your back and head have to create an absolutely straight line during Palming. If you are doing it from work in front of the computer, place your elbows on the desk, and then place your head into prepared palms. If your head is bent down then move the chair back from the desk and bend over until your back and your neck create a straight line. The reason is that the major blood vessels and spinal cord must not be curved during relaxation.

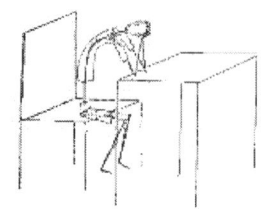

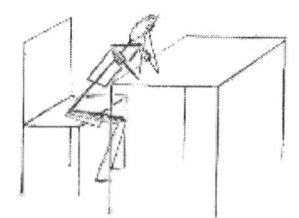

Chapter 5 – Acupressure

Let's take a break and boost some energy into the eye area. The best way is a Shiatsu method which is also called Acupressure. 'Shiatsu' is Japanese for 'pressuring by finger'. The force of the massaging finger is applied to the same dots that are used by acupuncture. The science of acupressure and acupuncture dates back many centuries. There are many different ideas about how this method was born. One of them talks about a Chinese soldier that had a stiff shoulder, which was very uncomfortable and painful. The doctor in the soldier's village could not do anything to help the poor fellow. Then the soldier was called to war, and one day when he was fighting in a battle, his leg was pierced by an enemy's arrow. The soldier bent down to retrieve the arrow's tip out of his leg, and suddenly he noticed that the constant pain in his shoulder was gone. I am not too sure if the enemy became an instant friend right away, but when the soldier returned home, he told the doctor all about his miraculous healing.

This is just one of the many stories about the way the method of acupuncture was born. Acupuncture is popular and has been practiced in Japan, China, India, Korea, Vietnam and Siberia dating back to the Stone Age.

There have been ancient books discovered that have diagrams of the meridians and the acupuncture points located along these meridians. The human body has different systems of circulation built in that either flow internally or socialize with the Universe. For example, your heart pushes blood through your arteries and veins to various organs and muscles. The respiratory system is used when we inhale air, pass oxygen to the blood and brain, then we exhale and pass it out to the atmosphere. The digestive system transforms food that we eat into nutrients that our bodies need to build cells.

Take a look at the picture that displays Digestive, Respiratory, Nervous and Lymphatic systems:

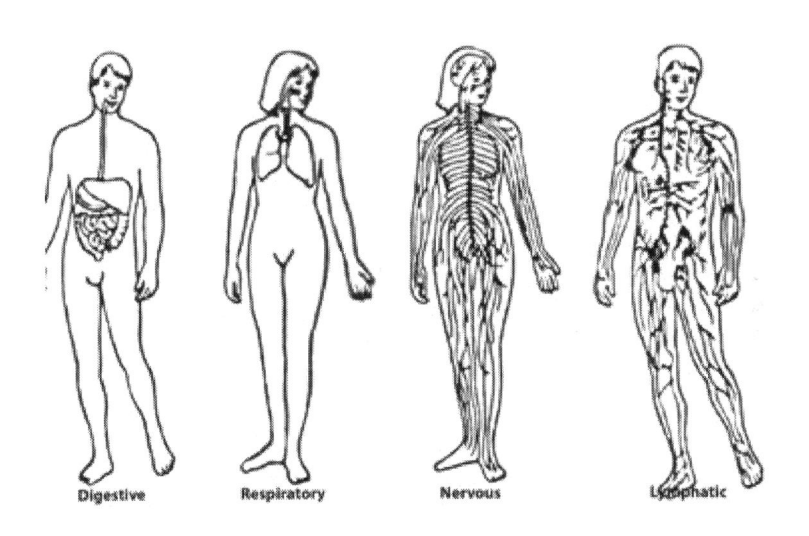

Digestive   Respiratory   Nervous   Lymphatic

Just imagine how much sorting has to be done while the digestive system 'looks' at the food we supply to our body and identifies what is essential, and what has to be eliminated as excess and unnecessary.

Meridians are pathways used for energy throughout the body. If there is something wrong with an organ or muscle, they pass this information along to the meridian responsible for that organ or muscle.

Below is the picture of meridians.

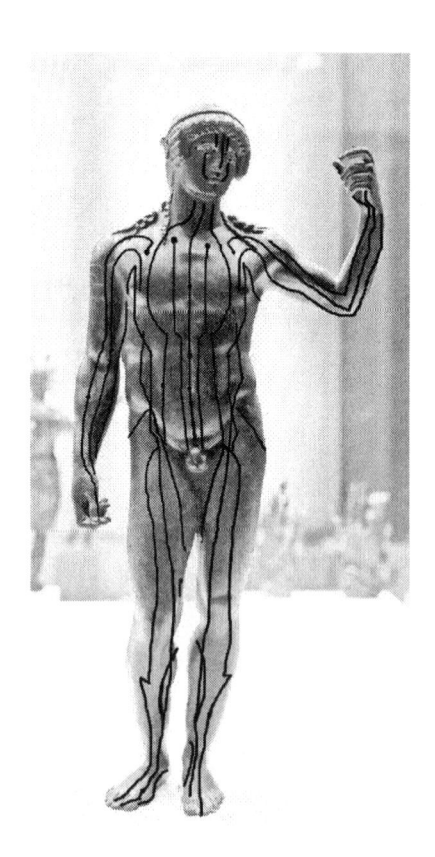

The meridian is then going to send a signal through certain points (spots) on the body. These spots will become painful, crying out for help. If their screams are noticed quickly, then the illness can be prevented before it starts to affect the body. By simply massaging these screaming dots or inserting an acupuncture needle, it is possible to restore the energy flow and thus correct the problem of the corresponding organ or muscle.

I am not suggesting that you use acupuncture needles - you should only see a professional acupuncturist - but we can simply follow a few shiatsu rules in order to perform a professional eye massage on ourselves.

To Begin Eye Acupressure

Use either the tip of the middle finger or the knuckle of the same finger.

If you use the tip of your finger, make sure that your nails do not cut the skin of the massaged area. Do not bend your finger.

Ways of applying pressure

GOOD   BAD   BAD

Use spiral or circular movements. Do not move your finger (or knuckle) back and forth.

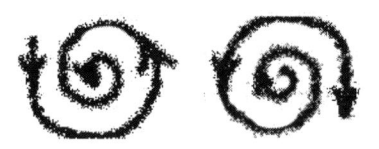

Eye Acupressure Points

The first dot is located at both sides of the bridge of your nose. Find the spot that reacts with the pain on the finger pressure.

Use your middle finger tips to press to this point.

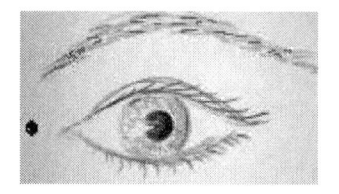

During this little massage exercise, you will find that your eyesight will become much better, especially when you press on the dot from both sides of your nose.

The next dot is located right underneath your pupils. Work on it for a minute, using different pressures by the massaging fingers.

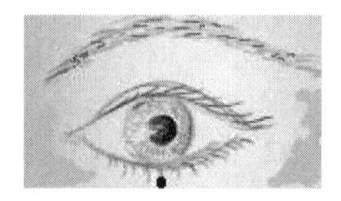

Then the next points will be your temple.

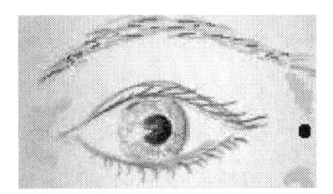

You have to remember these dots are either painful or feel like there is a hole in the bone (do not use any other objects for pressure on these dots except your own fingers).

The last point of pressure (and usually the most painful) is located in the middle of the eyebrow.

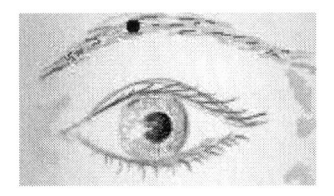

In addition, you may add two more important points that are also located on the eyebrows.

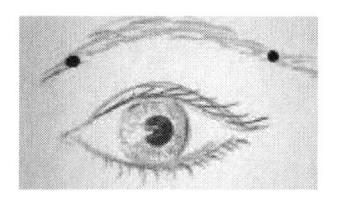

The meridians in our body are not the organ's only map - there are many others that could be used for diagnosis and treatments. You may find the condition of your health displayed on your tongue, your palms, nails, face, feet, ears and the irises of your eyes.

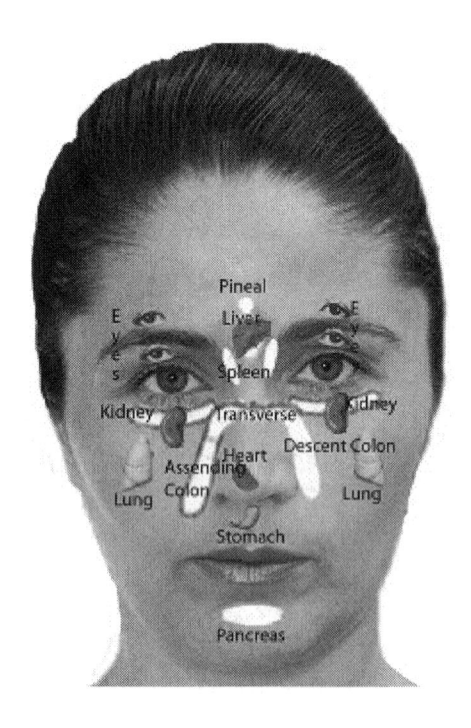

For diagnosis only, irises and the tongue are used as pictures of your body's condition, but palms, fingers, feet and ears display the health status as well as transferring received energy that is being applied by the finger pressure.

Picture of Ear Chart

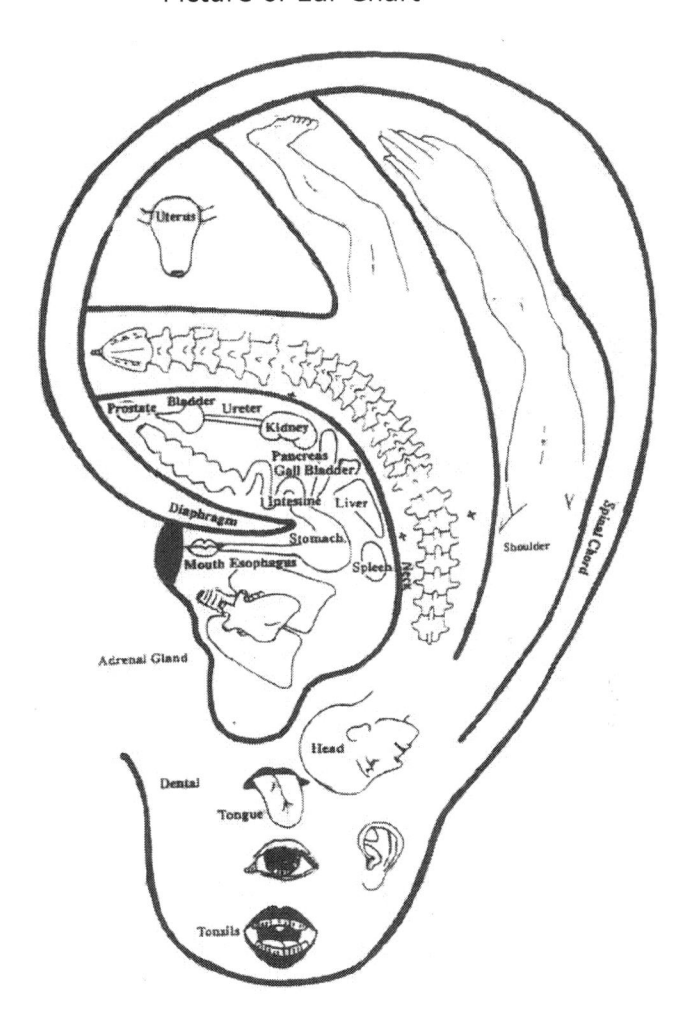

   Therefore, finding hurting points on your feet, ears, fingers and palms, and massaging them until the triggered zones become soft and less painful, will certainly help the whole body to relieve pain, release stress from the muscles and a faster return to better health.

Picture of Feet Chart

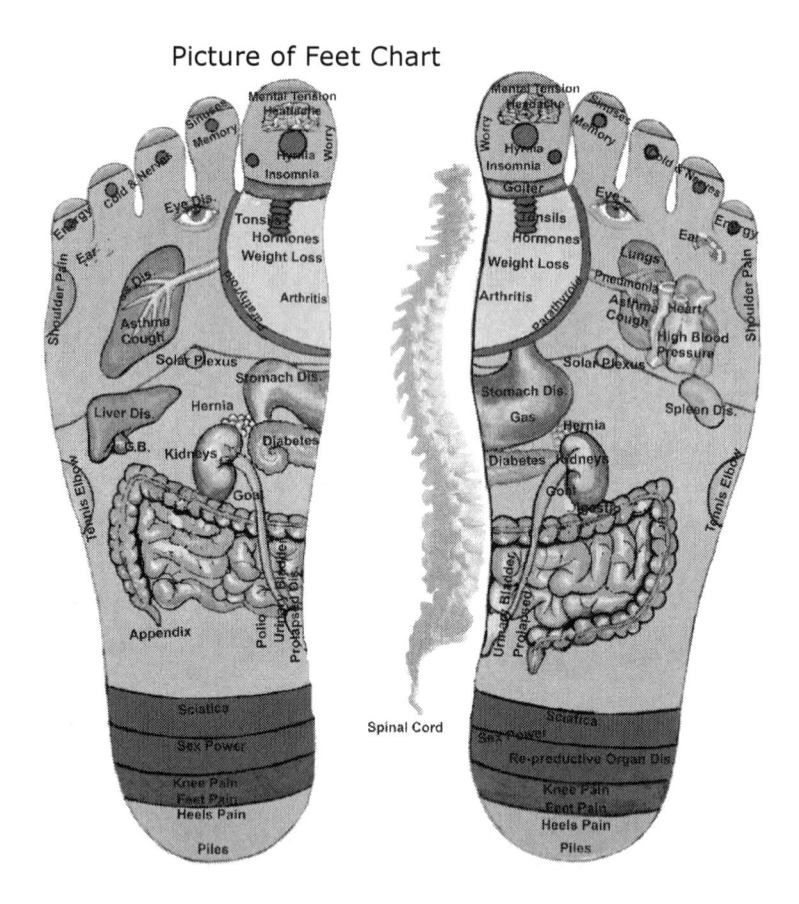

Apparently, Eastern medicine schools show a relationship between the organ's condition and how the eyeball moves. For example, the doctor will ask the patient to look left or right, up and down, or, which is the most important, a full circle by your eyes. If during drawing circles the patient cuts off any corners, the doctor will immediately translate what is not working perfectly in the patient's body. By the analogy of the direct connection between acupuncture points and your organs, you can make a conclusion by eye movements (especially when drawing the circles). The conclusion is that when you are trying to make perfect circles with your eyes. you are also forcing your inner body parts to function perfectly too.

Picture of Right Iris Chart

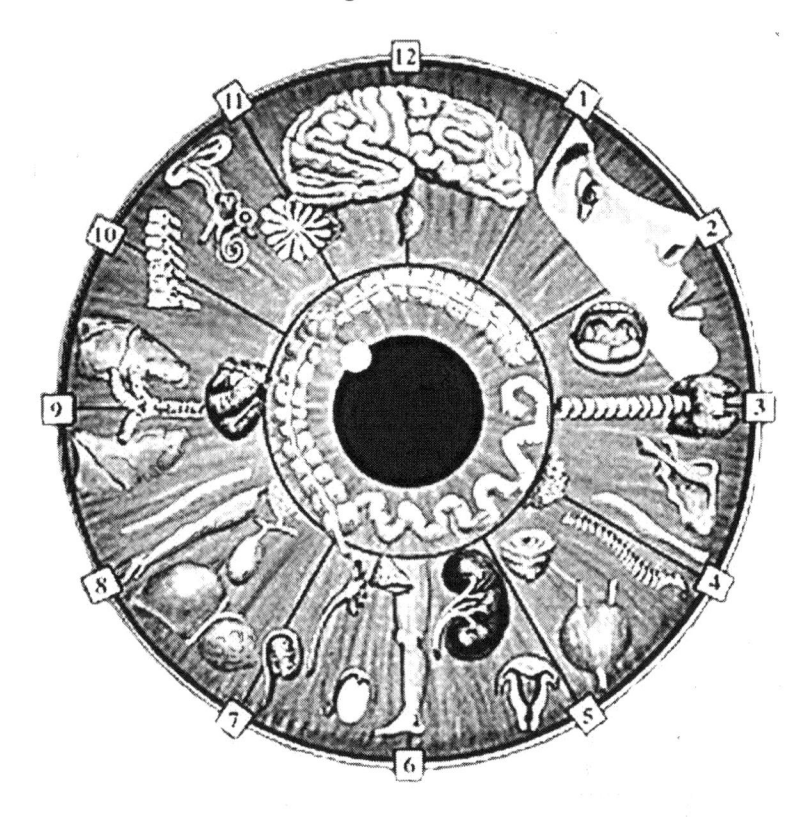

But let's return to our eye exercises. Close your eyes and try to relax for a few moments.

Now you are ready for the next set of exercises.

Chapter 6 – Dynamic Set

Please remember to keep your back straight, your stomach in, your chest out, and your chin up. Always check your position.

Actually, let's check to make sure your posture is correct. Find a straight wall in the place where you are right now and stand against it. If you have the perfect posture that I am talking about from the beginning of this book, the body parts that touch the wall in this moment are:

 - your heels,
 - your calves,
 - your buttocks,
 - your shoulder blades,
 - the back of your head

Now try to keep this posture while you walk around the room. Do it very slowly in the beginning. Walk straight along one of the walls in the room, turn around and then come back to the same wall where you had that wonderful transformation. If all of the body parts that I listed are touching the wall after your walk around the room, then you are ready to continue.

While you are standing (or sitting) in the newly-learned perfect posture position, glance to the most left position, then quickly glance to the most right position and return back to the left. Repeat 7 - 8 times. Keep up the speed. Follow up with blinking.

The eye movements now have to begin from the far right position going to the far left. Make sure you are doing absolute straight lines with your eyes. Repeat 7 - 8 times. Follow up with blinking.

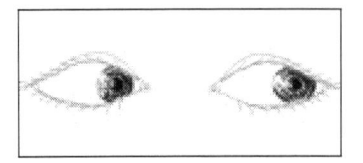

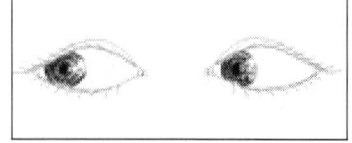

Then roll your eyes up to the sky (ceiling). Quickly look down to your feet and return your gaze back up again. Repeat 7 - 8 times. Follow up with blinking. Your chin should not move during these movements.

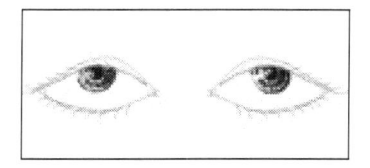

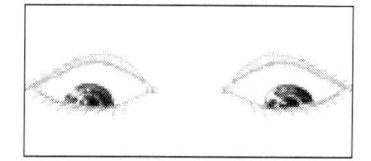

Now begin with looking down at your feet and then look up to the sky and return back down. Complete 7 - 8 straight lines. Follow up with blinking.

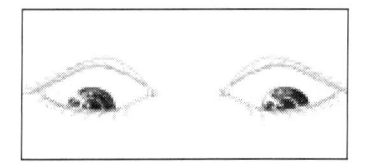

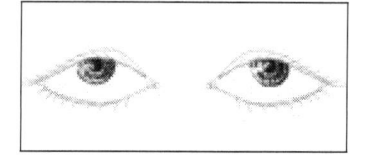

Now make the diagonal moves - begin with the top left corner and look down to the right corner and then to the left upper corner. After repeating it for 7 - 8 times, relax your eyes with blinking. Now repeat in the opposite direction. And as before, relax your eyes with blinking.

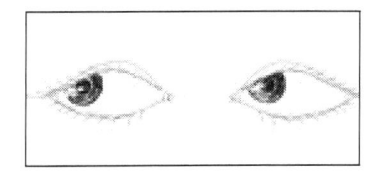

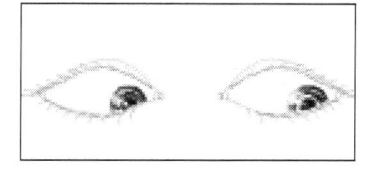

Now for another combination – right top corner to the left bottom corner in both directions. Complete 7 – 8 straight lines. Follow up with blinking.

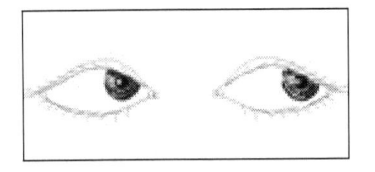

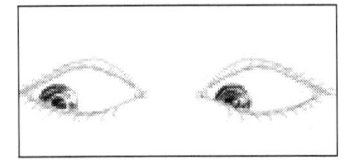

It does not matter what kind of blinking you perform – either butterfly blinking or blind blinking (with eyes closed) or even hard blinking that brings out tears almost right away. Just follow with the type that you feel is the best for you at this particular moment.

Go back to the wall, check your posture, inhale, and at the same time you inhale, stretch up like you are trying to grow, and, after exhaling (but keeping up the perfect posture) let's make some advanced movements:

1. Roll your eyes up to the upper right corner, and then quickly look down to the right bottom corner and up to the upper right corner again.

   Repeat 5 - 7 times and blink-blink-blink-blink.

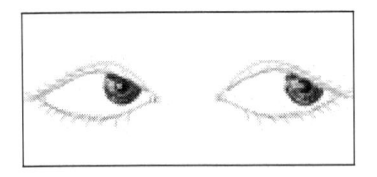

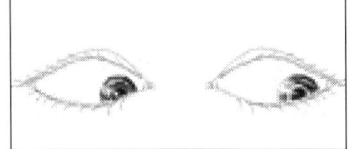

   Repeat in the opposite direction – from the right bottom corner to the right upper corner and back to the right bottom corner. It is very important to make the lines as straight as possible.

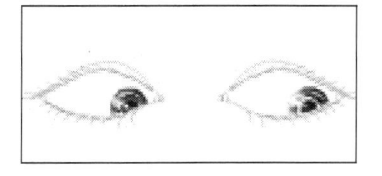

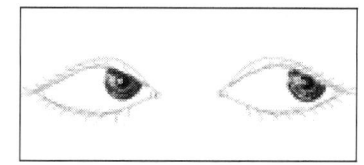

2. Now draw the line on the bottom - look at the bottom right corner (your right shoulder), glance over to the bottom left corner (your left shoulder) and back to the bottom right corner. Repeat a few times and finish up with blinking.

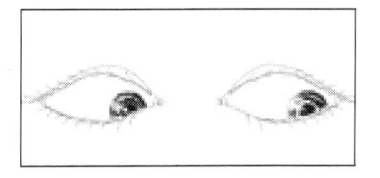

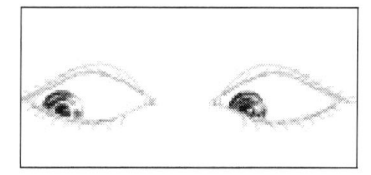

3. The next line will be on your left side – from the left bottom corner to the upper left and back. Proceed with the same technique, and finish up with blinking.

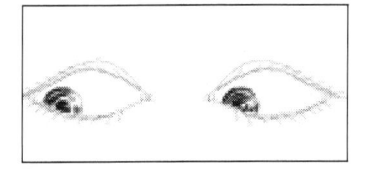

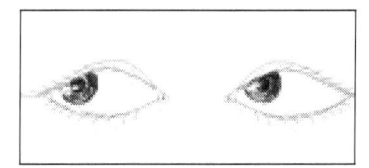

4. And the last one is the upper line – from the upper left corner to the upper right corner and back. Finish up with blinking.

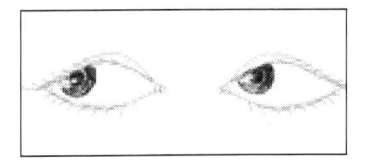

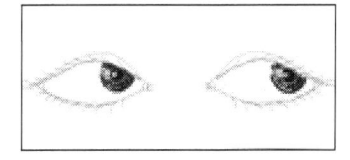

Little tip: I try to make all the eye exercises interesting. In the case of the Dynamic Set, I use objects that are located around my workplace. For example, for the right bottom corner I would look at the phone. I would use the orchid's flowers as left upper corner. Just place different objects around you in the manner that will suit your own purpose and use the location of these objects.

Fun part: Try to draw an alphabet with your eyes.
Repeat the Dynamic Set with closed eyes and finish with blind blinking.

Chapter 7 – In Case of Emergency

Despite all the precautions that you may take, your eyes may still hurt from time-to-time. That proves that you still did not learn how to relax your eyes. Here are some techniques that you can use to either calm the pain down or prevent its appearance:

Method 1 - Contrast Eye Bathing

I simplified this procedure to a bare minimum. When I feel that my upper eyelids are puffy and red, and the skin under my eyebrows is sagging down, I grab one piece of ice (any size) and stand beside something hot (a tap with running hot water or a sink filled with hot water, making sure it does not burn your skin). Ensure that the ice cube does not stick to your skin (just rub it against your hand first), then make a few circles over your closed eyes with this piece of ice and right away, splash your closed eyes with the hot water (careful though! Do not boil your eyes, you may still need them!).

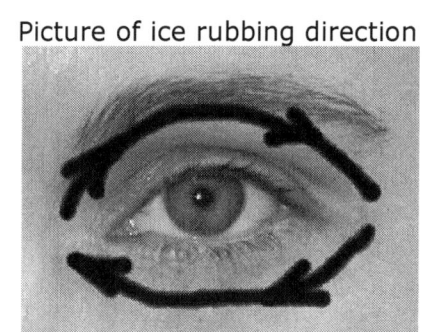

Picture of ice rubbing direction

Repeat this 7 - 8 times and all of the puffiness will disappear. This procedure can also be used by women anytime to revitalize their eyes.

Variations of this procedure:

- Instead of splashing hot water on your face, you can use a cotton pad that you soaked in hot water.
- If you do not want to deal with an ice cube, then just use a cotton pad after you soaked it in a bowl filled with very cold water.
- And remember that it is very important that in this procedure, you start with cold and finish with cold.

Method 2 – Tea Cotton Pads

If you have loose tea leaves in your home, you can do the following: make very strong tea (1 teaspoon in ¼ cup hot water), steep for 3 - 5 minutes and strain. I personally prefer black tea (without any additives or flavours) for this procedure. Place your hot tea either outside (only if it is colder than inside) or in the fridge for a few minutes. When the tea cools down, soak some cotton pads in this tea, lie down on a bed (floor, sofa) without a pillow and place these soaked pads on your closed upper eyelids. The temperature of the tea is totally an individual preference. Experiment with applying warm or cold tea-soaked cotton pads on your eyes and find out what is the most comfortable temperature for you.

Method 3 – Complete Relaxation

Lie down, close your eyes, and let them take the most comfortable position in the eye sockets. Then relax. Imagine black space in front of you. Do nothing, and continue to relax to the point where you stop feeling your eyes in your eye sockets. And then spread the relaxation down to the whole body. Relax all of the face muscles: the ones around your eyes, then temple muscles, then cheeks, mouth, upper jaws, and chin. Make sure that your upper row of teeth is not pressing down on the lower row. Finish up with the forehead and the back of your head.

Now push down this relaxation feeling to the throat, back of your neck, shoulders, upper arms, elbows, wrists, palms and fingers. The arms become heavy; they are soft, warm and very heavy. Continue with the torso, then going down to the waist, pelvis, and buttocks. Push the relaxation further down to both legs – thighs, knees, shins and finish up with your heels and toes. If any unwanted thoughts come into your mind at this moment, just smile at them from inside without moving a single muscle on your face and let them go peacefully. You will be able to come back to these thoughts later and think them through when you finish the exercising.

All of the relaxation methods can be used at any time of the day. If you finish the exercises earlier then you expected, top them up with a few relaxing methods (palming, staring at nothing, closed eyes and looking at black space, full relaxation of the whole body, etc.).

Chapter 8 – Focusing Exercises

This set is a real pleasure to perform after the warm up you have just completed. But before you jump into this exciting routine, you need to gain an understanding of the core idea. We need to make the eyes able to see objects that are close in the same way as objects in the distance (for the far sighted) and vise versa (for the near sighted). Find an item that is always with you and small enough in that it is a kind of abstract dot. I usually use the tip of my nail on an index finger. Hold it in front of you in the most comfortable position for your eyes distance (meaning that you are able to see all of the little details clearly from this distance). Now slowly start moving your finger closer to the tip of your nose, keeping your attention on the nail tip while trying to see all of the details in the same clear manner.
Closer….
    Closer…..

When it is impossible to look at the fingertip without seeing the edges of the nail tip sharp and clear, glance far away to relax the eye muscles and return your finger into the starting position.

Now try to do this again, but instead of moving your finger closer and closer to your nose, do this in the opposite direction – start moving it further and further, then return your finger back to the original position.

Now that you understand the logic of this focusing exercise, you can begin to complete it again, but using one eye at a time.

1. Cover up your better-seeing eye with your palm (just make sure that the inner part of the palm does not touch the upper eyelid) and begin doing the exercise described above. If both your eyes have the same prescription, than it does not matter which eye you begin with. Complete about 8 - 10 movements for each eye (moving your finger slowly back and fourth, keeping perfect focusing on the details of the fingernail tip).

2. Change the direction of your moving finger. Instead of moving it back and fourth, move it to the left until it is impossible to see the fingernail details (by the way, the posture still has to be perfect and your head cannot move with your eyes). From the most left position, move your finger to the most right position, keeping focused on your uncovered eye of the moving finger. Perform 8 - 10 movements and continue with the eye that was covered before.
Relax your eyes with blinking and repeat this exercise with both eyes open.

3. Move your finger diagonally. Follow the finger with your eyes. Repeat first with the eye that sees worse and keep the "better" eye covered. Then perform exactly the same procedure but cover the eye that has just performed the exercise. Please remember to maintain good posture!

4. With one eye covered, move your finger to the most comfortable spot for the eye position (usually it is 30-33 cm, but it depends on your eyes' condition). Focus your gaze on your index fingernail tip, then change your focus to the tip of your nose, then back to the fingernail tip. Make sure that both of these objects (nail and the tip of your nose) are on the same visualized line, meaning that you do not need to move your eyesight left or right, you have to change your focus only. Repeat 10 times and follow up with blinking. Open the covered eye, cover your other eye and complete the same set of focusing changes. Relax your eyes with blinking.

5. Look around and choose an object that is located at least a few feet away (a tree in the window, traffic light, pool, etc.) and focus your eyesight on that object. Then change your focus to the tip of your nose. Repeat 8 - 10 times. Remember that all of the objects that you focus on have to be on the same line. Cover your other eye and repeat this exercise in exactly the same manner.

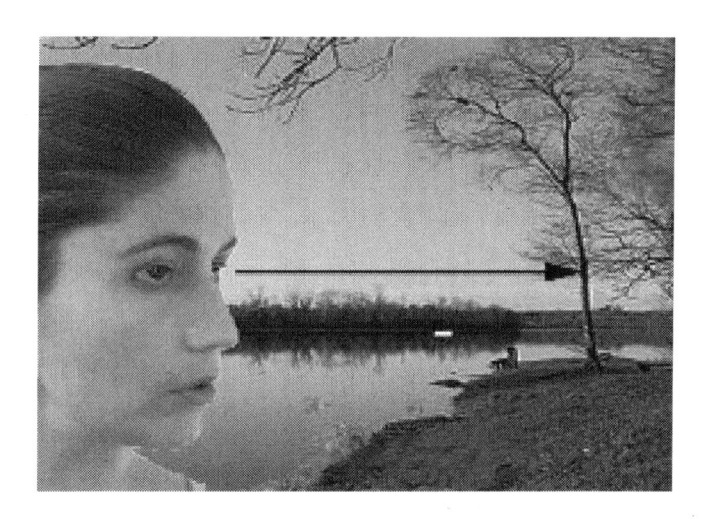

6. Focus on the tip of your nose, then on your finger, then at the furthest object and then do this in the opposite order (from a further object to your finger and then to your tip of your nose).

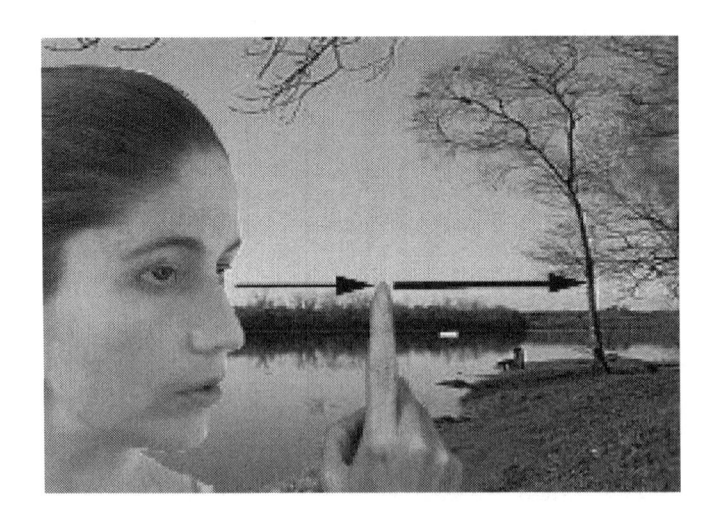

6. Try different variations of these focusing exercises. Try to perform focusing exercises whenever you have time. For example, while you are in the bus you can focus on electric polls that are on your way.

   Or, if you are driving, try to look at the speedometer and then at the road further ahead. When you go for a walk in the park, look at a tree that is close to you and then glance to a tree that is further away.

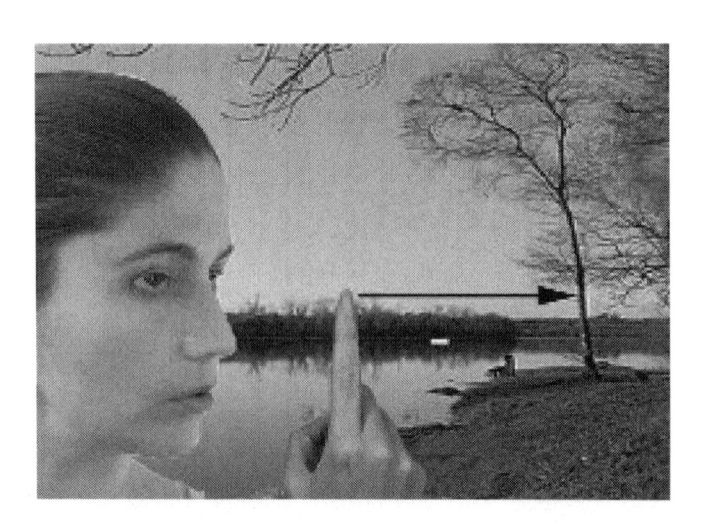

When you finish all of the exercises, complete them with any relaxation technique or splash your eyes with cold water (if there is a chance to do so).

Chapter 9 – Watching the Sun

At the beginning of writing this book, my intention was to create a simple and practical handbook that would include eye exercises themselves without any explanation of their history. But later, during interactions with different people during my lectures, I realized that giving just the physical side of this complex process of restoring vision is not enough. We tend to succeed with greater results when we know what is behind the idea. That is why I decided to give you a few descriptions that would give an obvious reason why we do certain types of eye exercises.

Let's compare plants that grow in a greenhouse and the same kinds of plants that grow outside and receive the full spectrum of nature's conditions – real sunlight, oxygen with a wind that always brings different particles from neighboring plants and trees, different amounts of humidity, insects, bees, and so on. The plants with a greenhouse atmosphere will still be green, but compared to the ones that grow outside, these indoor plans will have weak trunks, thinner leaves, and their quality will be at least 10 times lower that the quality of the ones that grew outside. Now, let's imagine that we decided to tone the glass of our greenhouse. For some ridiculous reason we decided that too much sun is going to damage the weak plants. But, interestingly, we are getting opposite results – our plants are dying. I hope you understand this. Let's compare our sunglasses to toned glass of that greenhouse.

The Sun gives our eyes a true power that nothing else can give. Sunlight is absolutely necessary for improving the blinking and tearing process. The Sun helps our eyes restore the moisture level and become shiny, which give our eyes life. It is never too late to learn the procedures of sun watching. Use it whenever you can.

Start by doing swing turns with your eyes closed. You can also simply turn your head from left to right and from right to left. Let the Sun's rays give its energy directly to your upper eyelids. Follow up with palming.

Close your eyes and turn your head to the sun. Begin by placing your palms on your closed eyes and then taking them off. Kids call this "Peek-a-boo".

The only time when direct sun-watching is recommended is either at sunrise or sunset, when the sun is not extremely bright. Stand up straight, covering one eye with your palm. Watch the sun for as long as you can without blinking, or until the tears start coming out of your eye and it will be unbearable to continue. Then cover this eye with your palm and perform exactly the same procedure with the other eye. You have to look right at the center of the sun and try to make the sun fill up the entire space in front of you. Hint: When you are watching the sun, think that its flame is gently cleaning your eyes, washing them, and giving energy all at the same time.

A Little History

Apparently, there are people in this world that live on the sun's energy. They are called sun-eaters. These people charge themselves from the sun like they are live batteries.

Just the idea of looking at the sun without any barriers makes you think that it is an absolutely crazy idea. In the beginning, you will not be able to look at the sun for more then just a few seconds. Then, if you continue watching it from day to day (except a rainy or snowy day), you will find that you are able look longer and longer.

Whenever you perform sun-watching procedures, finish them up with Palming. The time you spend Palming should be at least twice as long as the watching procedure itself.

Chapter 10 – Observations from My Experience

All of the exercises I have written about in this book I have practiced on myself. I'm going to share with you now a few observations that I have made during this process.

Observation 1 – Sun-Watching

I have found out that watching the sunrise appears to be a truly enjoyable experience, and noticed that if I was able to see even the short appearance of the sun rising in the morning, the rest of the day will be as beautiful as the sun in the sunrise! Nothing will be able to spoil the rest of the day.

Observation 2 – Binocular Effect

There is a very interesting effect that appears right at the beginning of eye exercising. I call this the "binocular effect" because it feels like somebody suddenly adjusts the lenses in the binoculars. This effect is noticeable only when you do not wear glasses and it becomes more and more frequent and each time it lasts longer.

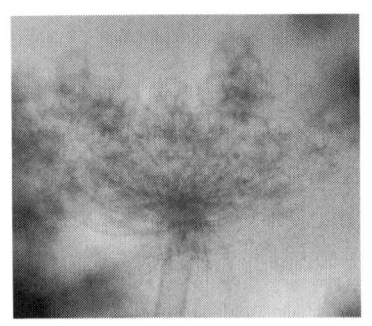

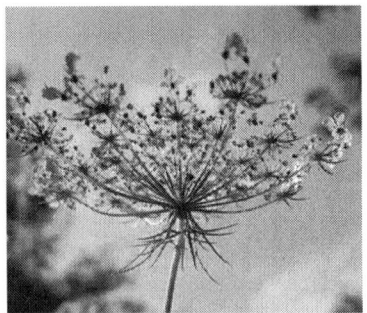

With the first few occurrences, this effect lasts just before the next blink of your eyes. Then you are able to hold on to this condition beyond 3 - 4 blinks and longer. It also lasts longer and occurs more often when it is cold out, somewhere outside of the city, or walking in the park. The only explanation I came up with was the fact that the air is much cleaner in the winter, in the suburbs, and in park areas.

Therefore, THE MOST IMPORTANT RULE is TAKE YOUR GLASSES OFF and make your eye muscles work! If your eyes get extremely tired, just do any of the relaxing parts of eye exercising – either do very fast blinking, hard blinking, blinking with closed eyes, palming, contrast eye bathing, or tea dipping. I understand that sometimes getting rid of your glasses completely is absolutely impossible (for example, for the person that needs to drive everyday). In this case, I came up with an idea - just buy glasses with a smaller prescription. You may experience a little challenge in this direction. Most of the eyewear shops require a doctor's prescription and they will never, under any circumstances make a pair of glasses that is 1 diopter lower than your current prescription. Please be patient with the sales people. They are very sensitive to their product and will defend the idea that glasses and contact lenses are the only perfect way to correct your vision.

In order not to harm your own neurological system, under any circumstances DO NOT TRY to prove them otherwise, even if you have already have unprecedented improvement with your vision. I am trying to warn you because I have been in a situation where one sales person (he was wearing glasses) started shouted at me when he found out the reason why I wanted to get glasses with a lower prescription. I ran out of the store and burst into tears, thinking that all of my improvements are just temporary and my vision will return back to the very, very, bad condition it was in before I started these experiments. And I gave up...

I stopped doing my exercises.

I fell into depression.

But then a few months later, I noticed that the glasses I was wearing were already two diopters down from the original prescription and the glasses that I was wearing before are really too strong for me and I cannot go back to them. Then, a few weeks later, I needed to do some curtain sewing and I accidentally noticed that I am doing it WITHOUT my glasses and I can easily concentrate on the needle's ear!!! I used to have a bad astigmatism problem and I was not able to concentrate in the middle of the reading table that optometrists use for evaluation of the eyesight. Well, these two stable results talked for themselves.

I thought that one day I will come back to that sales person and demonstrate to him my perfect vision. But now, I don't even want to bother because I gained an understanding why this person was vocal to me. He was just simply defending his zone of comfort, his own reality where people are not responsible for their own eyes! He seems to believe that he is not able to change anything about his health and that there are circumstances around him that brought him to this condition and the only help is a doctor's prescription. But when this person finds out that there is something else out there that only he is responsible for, he will have to make a choice and he will have to make it by himself – either to abandon his own health (in this case - eyes) and do nothing or take responsibility.

There are many people that live their life and prefer that somebody else make decisions for them and then they blame that somebody for the decisions they made about their life. They blame doctors that did not heal them, they blame the teachers that did not teach them, they blame the employers that did not care enough about them and they definitely blame the government for any possible reason! Just keep away from these kinds of people. They are sick with the illness that I call BRAINolaziya. And this sickness is extremely contagious! If you are affected by this illness, the symptoms are as following: temporary depressions, moodiness, low level of energy, no smile, bouquet of illnesses, and so on....

But, let's go back to my observation experience.

Observation 3 – Listen to your body

I also noticed that when you are sick (with a cold, pulled muscle, etc.) you do not feel like doing eye exercises. This feeling is the voice of your smart body telling you that exercising your eyes will not bring any results at this time. I would suggest you take care of the immediate situation and, when you get better, return to exercising your eyes again. Do not worry - the new vision will not worsen, it will stay where you left it. But I would suggest you keep up with nutrition that is good for your eyes.

Observation 4 – Mind Adjustment

Interestingly, I found out about the ability of our mind to take a certain amount of time in order to get used to the adjustments that are happening in our body. For example, after a week of eye exercises you find out that you can read at a further distance than before, but you also notice that your hands still hold the reading material at the previous distance when your vision was worse! And you have to adjust all of your habits to a new vision. It looks like the mind is still holding on to your previous habits and is not letting your body adjust to the new improvements until it gets used to it.

Here is the diagram and how it works:

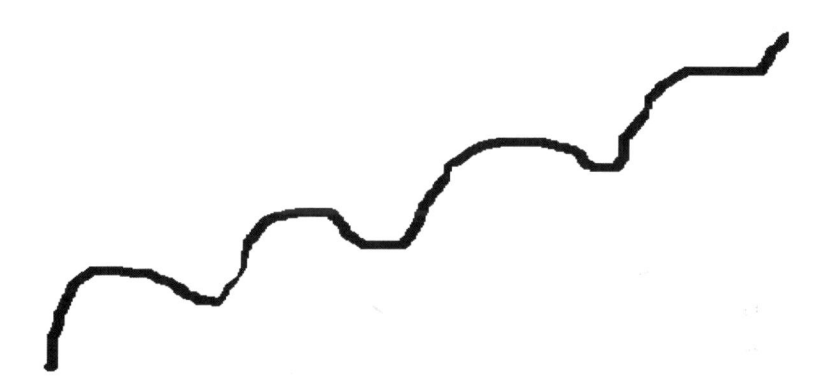

It could be the fluctuation of your vision's condition during one session. It could also be a month of eye exercises. Your vision may change during the same day, but you will only notice it when you do not have your glasses on. But, despite any of the harmful effects, you are still improving!

Observation 5 – Positive Side Effects

Apparently, there are a few side effects that you may notice when you perform eye exercises for awhile. They are related to multiple face muscles twitching. I used to have this twitching appear in my eyebrow, upper and bottom eyelids and the top of one of my cheeks. Thankfully, these face muscle movements were not happening at the same time, but whenever any of them occurred, I felt really embarrassed. I thought that everybody noticed my condition. Unfortunately, I cannot say exactly after what period of time of doing eye exercises all of these twitches disappeared, but it was not long.

Part 3

Chapter 1 - Nutrition

We are what we eat – there is nothing new about that! Scientific research and the experience of generations show your eyes need Vitamins A, B, C and E included in your diet every day.

A Carrot juice
  Kale
  Broccoli leaves
  Tomatoes
  Sweet potatoes
  Spinach
  Melon, cantaloupe, honey dew
  Peas
  Lettuce
  Green onions
  Pumpkin

B	Potatoes
	Bananas
	Lentils
	Green leafy vegetables
	Asparagus
	Broccoli
C	Rose hips
	Black Current
	Red Pepper
	Red Current
	Brussels sprouts
	Lychee
	Papaya
	Mango
	Pickled cabbage
	Citrus (any)
D	Sunshine
	Pine nuts
	Royal jelly

The best way to consume these products is in their raw form without any thermo processing, which can tremendously reduce the amount of vitamins.

Don't be afraid to experiment in the kitchen! Just try to mix up some vegetables and fruits together and you will definitely come up with some new art form of vitamin-rich salads!

Here are a few recipes that are extremely helpful during Eye Exercising. All of the products in these recipes must be organic and in their raw condition.

Chapter 2 – Recipes

Here are a few recipes that will help introduce you to a "living on live food" diet (raw food). These recipes are specifically designed for your eye needs.

Recipe 1 – Beet and Zucchini Salad

Ingredients:

1 Young Zucchini, shredded
1 Carrot, shredded
¼ Red Onion, diced
½ cup Parsley, chopped
1 Beet, shredded
½ Lemon, juiced
Sea salt to taste
Black pepper to taste
1 tablespoon olive oil

Shred carrot, beet and zucchini. Dice the onion. Mix all the ingredients in a large salad bowl and then add the chopped parsley. Whisk in the lemon juice, add sea salt and black pepper to taste, then add the olive oil. Variations: you can also add snow peas if they are available. Top up the dish with sesame seeds.

Recipe 2 – Chickpea Salad

Ingredients:

5 - 6 Radishes
1 Pickle
1 cup of Alfalfa sprouts
1/3 cup of fresh Dill, chopped
1/3 cup of fresh Parsley, chopped
1/3 cup of Chickpeas (soaked overnight)
½ cup of Kale, shredded
Sea salt
Black pepper
2 tablespoons Olive Oil or Grapeseed Oil

Soak the Chickpeas overnight. In the morning, rinse them and add more fresh water. Drain just before you are ready to make the salad. Cut the radishes in half and slice them. Cut the pickle in half lengthwise and then slice it also. Chop the fresh dill and parsley, and add the shredded kale. Add sea salt and black pepper to taste. Mix everything up, sprinkle with olive oil and top with alfalfa sprouts.

Recipe 3 – Raw Carrot Soup

Ingredients:

3 cups fresh carrot juice
1 Tablespoon light miso paste
½ tsp Bragg's Liquid Aminos
1 small clove garlic, crushed (or ¼ tsp garlic powder)
2 tsp fresh basil (or ½ tsp dried crushed basil)
1 avocado, peeled, seeded and diced
2 ears sweet corn, husked (and kernels removed from cob)
1 Tablespoon minced red onion
1 Tablespoon fresh cilantro, chopped

Put the carrot juice, miso, Braggs, garlic powder, and basil in a blender. Add half the avocado, the tomatoes and corn kernels, and puree. Combine the remaining vegetables, except cilantro, and toss. To serve, pour pureed mixture into individual bowls and stir in tossed vegetables. Serve chilled, at room temperature, or warmed to 115 degrees. Garnish with cilantro.

Recipe 4 – Spinach Salad

Salad Ingredients:

1 cup of Spinach, chopped
1 cup of Cherry Tomatoes
½ cup of Wild leek (if unavailable, substitute with ¼ cup of chopped chives)
 Dressing Ingredients:

½ cup of soaked almonds
6 leaves of spinach
1 teaspoon of organic mustard

1 tablespoon of olive oil
2 tablespoons of mineral water
Sea salt to taste
Black pepper to taste

Preparation (does not take more than 5 min.):

Put all of the Dressing ingredients into a food processor and chop it for a minute.

Mix spinach and tomatoes, then add some chopped wild leek (if possible). Pour dressing over the salad and enjoy!

Chapter 3 – Herbal Medicine

Herbal medicine is the oldest form of healthcare known to man. Herbs have been used by all cultures throughout history. During my research on Herbal Medicine for Eye Health, I was able to find information about a few types of berries that were used for centuries in different countries.

The first herb is called Chinese Schizandra Berry (Magnolia Vine) which grows in East Asia and Mongolia. It is mentioned in the early medical texts of China as one of the "superior herbs". Schizandra is capable of promoting good mental function in some aspects of learning and memory. It may also elevate your mood and is ideal if you are suffering from a lack of energy and nervous exhaustion from stress. Schizandra has traditionally been used to beautify the skin, strengthen blood vessels, and promote mental function and clarity. In Russia, Schizandra is a registered medicine for vision difficulties. You can either chew a pinch of dried berries (just don't eat the seeds, they don't taste good), or add 12 - 15 berries to your tea.

The other helpful type of berry used in herbal medicine is called Bilberry (Vaccinum myrtillus). The suggested daily dosage is either ¼ of a glass of freshly squeezed bilberry juice or 1 teaspoon of grinded berries mixed with ½ glass of water. This berry is famous for night vision improvement. Dried bilberry leaves make an exceptionally tasteful tea that is also good for the blood vessels of the eye.

People who suffer from myopia should take hawthorne with raw honey and eat it like jam. Use either fresh or dried hawthorne leaves to make a tea.

Carrot juice is extremely helpful, especially if you add 1 tablespoon of freshly squeezed parsley juice. Never overdo your intake of parsley juice. One tablespoon is the maximum. But you may safely add large quantities of parsley to your salads throughout the day.

Beet juice is excellent refreshment for the eyes (and for the whole body). You may even mix all three of them together – half a glass each of carrot and beet juice and 1 tablespoon of parsley juice.

Part 4

Chapter 1 – Posture and Spine Exercises

I hope you noticed that during all the different types of eye exercises, I meticulously repeat myself by reminding you to maintain perfect posture. Unfortunately, most of us do not know how important it is to keep our perfect posture, which really depends on the condition of the spine. In the Far East, people say "You are as Young as your Spine is Flexible". There are many reasons why I remind you throughout the book that during all types of Eye Exercises you have to keep the perfect posture while performing them. Only with the perfect posture will your brain and your eyes get the proper blood flow with the oxygen needed for muscle training and concentration. Proper energy flow is impossible without perfect posture. Even your emotions completely depend on your posture.

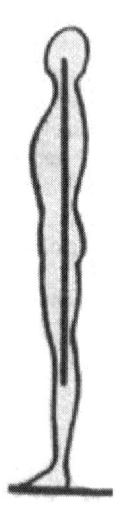

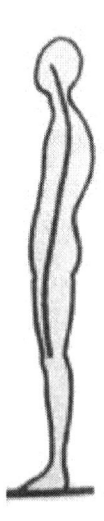

Let's conduct a simple experiment. Think about something really sad in your life - a time when you were upset, when you were about to cry, or when somebody was unfair to you (by your own opinion, of course!). When you get completely into the character, notice your posture, then notice the way your neck is bent forward, how your shoulders are rounded and how your chest hides inside.

As soon as all of the above mentioned positions for your body parts are noted, think about some funny moment in your life – something that made you laugh. Notice that suddenly your head goes up, your shoulders move behind and down, and your chest comes out of its hiding cave. As you can see, your overall health completely depends on your spine condition.

Let's learn a few easy spine stretching exercises that could be performed at home or at the workplace:

Exercise 1

Sit comfortably on a chair with your back straight. Your neck continues perfectly down the line of your back, shoulders back, chest out, stomach in. Place your palms on your thighs.

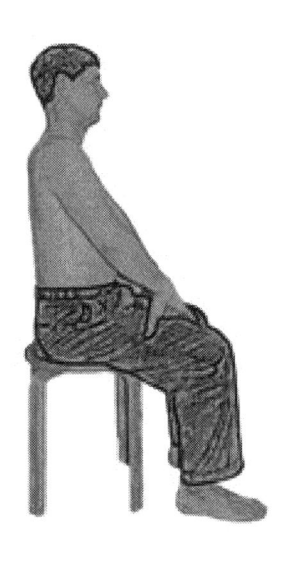

Inhale and push your palms down on your thighs and stretch your spine lengthwise, starting from the waist area and going up to the middle back, chest area and finally, to the neck. Do not look up - just stretch your neck by moving the crown of your head.

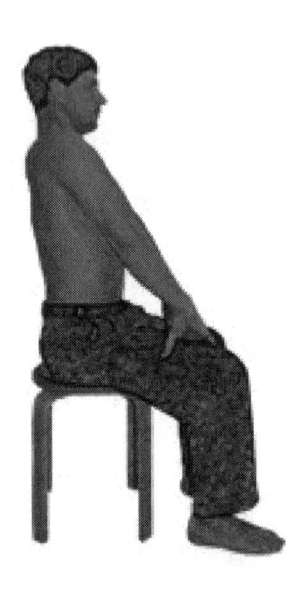

Exhale and keep this stretched position. With the next inhale, stretch more in exactly the same manner, beginning from the low part of your spine and ending up with the highest part of your neck. On the exhale, keep up with this stretched position.

And with the third inhale, try to stretch even more, following exactly the same technique described above. Then relax with an exhale, but do not bend your spine.

Exercise 2

Raise your arms up, rotating palms outward. The distance between your palms is a little larger than shoulder width.

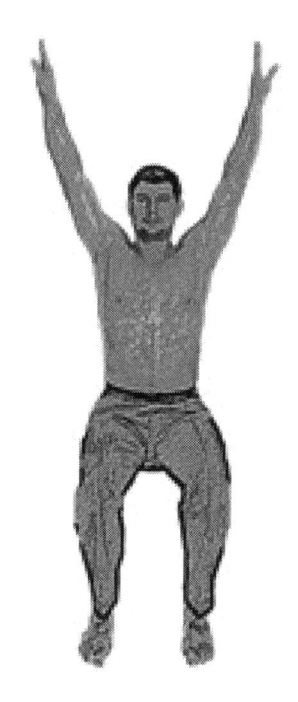

Lift your right shoulder to your right ear, stretching your spine.

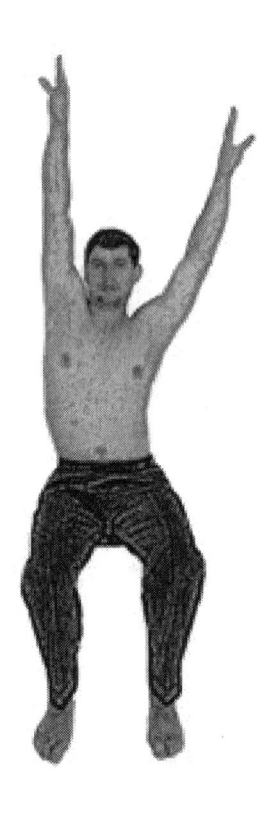

Don't tilt your head - keep your neck straight.

Repeat the same movement with your left shoulder and your left ear.

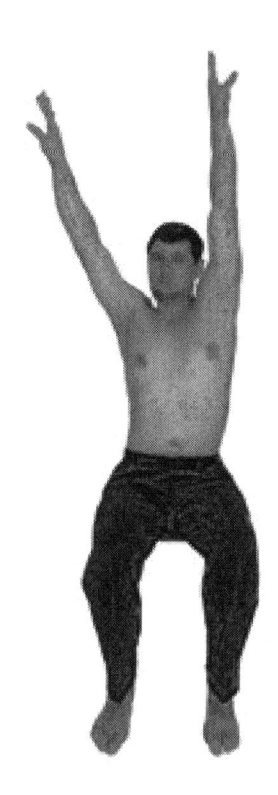

Chapter 2 – Eye Beauty

I used to be the woman that would have tons of eye make-up on to cover eye bags and dark circles under my eyes. Since I was squinting my eyes a lot in childhood, I got a few deep eye wrinkles even before I went to high school. I used very expensive creams, gels, and eye masks trying to improve my skin, but nothing was helping until during my eyesight improving research, I found a few extremely simple exercises for the muscles around the eyes. I placed all of these exercises into this chapter along with other simple tricks that will return the natural beauty back to your eyes.

- In the morning when you are about to wash your face, put some water into your mouth and splash ice-cold water onto your face. Perform this procedure anytime when you want your eyes to look instantly better.

- If you have puffy eyes, use either Contrast Eye Bathing that I described in the Emergency chapter or simply cut 2 slices of cucumber (organic) and place them for 15 – 20 minutes on your closed eyes while you are lying down without a pillow. Cucumber has natural ingredients to moisture the skin.

- In order to make your eyes shine bright, you have to work a little bit harder. There are a few stages involved to achieve this effect. First, massage all of your fingers from their tips to the base paying special attention to the smallest ones (pinkies). Then perform Acupressure massage as I described in the Acupressure chapter. When you are finished with the massage, go ahead to the final stage that I call 'hard blinking' (that is also considered an Eye Relaxation technique). Close your eyes as tight as possible, squeezing them as much as you can and then suddenly open them unexpectedly wide. Execute this type of blinking until the tears bust out of your eyes. As soon as this happens, your goal has been achieved. You also can use another trick - fill the sink with cold water and try to blink while your face is down in the water. The blood circulation tremendously speeds up inside of the tiny blood vessels of the eye at this moment, so please, do not get scared when you look at yourself in the mirror right at the end of this procedure!

Chapter 3 – Natural Eyelid Lifting

These face exercises improve the blood flow to the eye region, strengthen the upper and lower eyelids, and make bags under the eyes smaller or entirely disappear. The skin that used to hang over your eyes rises and is now toned, your eyebrows climb up, and by naturally pulling the skin you can increase your eyes' size. The appearance of your eyes becomes alive and attractive. It is suggested that you perform all of the exercises below twice a day during the first 10 days to see any visible reduction of the wrinkles.

Exercise 1

Place your middle fingers between the eyebrows above the bridge of your nose, and put your index fingers in the external corners of your eyes. Strain your lower eyelids and pull them upward. You need to feel how external eye muscles pulsate under your fingers. Strain your muscles even more, and then relax.

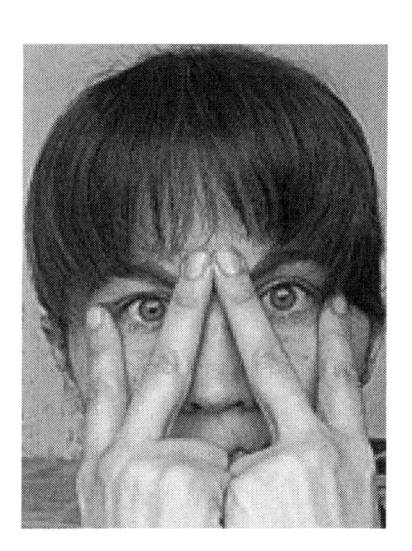

Repeat this exercise 10 times, concentrating your attention on your external eye muscles. After you have completed this 10 times, do not relax the lower eyelid muscles, but close your eyes and count to 40, still concentrating your attention on your external eye muscles. Do not relax while you count.

For the first 3 weeks, this exercise has to be performed at least twice a day. If the bags under your eyes are really big, then consider performing this exercise 3 times a day.

If you are in a hurry in the morning and have absolutely no time to complete this exercise, just make two repeats and then apply your makeup. The appearance of your eyes will be much better.

Exercise 2

Place two or three fingers on the bone that is located right below your eyes, gaze upwards and squint your bottom eyelids. Do not help yourself with your fingers; there are only eye muscles involved.

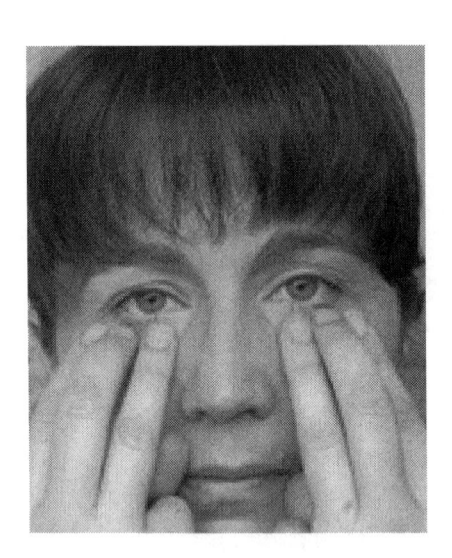

Repeat 10 times.

Perform the same exercise with your eyes closed, gazing upward. Repeat 10 times. And now we can repeat this exercise again while bending your head down.

End up with the EYE RELAXING Exercise that is called Palming.

Exercise 3 - Firming Upper Eyelids

Place your index fingers on your forehead right above the eyebrows and move them down. Try to pull up your eyebrows to the original position while your fingers are resisting. Relax all of your face muscles.

Repeat 10 times.

References

E.P. Yarozkaya, N. A. Fedorenko, E.V. Narishnaya "Eastern Methods of Healing", 1999, Moscow, ACT

Yog Ramanantata "Exercises for eyes", 2005, Grand

V. Vostokov "Secrets of Tibetian Medicine", 1997, St.Petersburg, KARO

A.Siderskiy, DVD "Introductory Course to Hatha-Yoga"

P.Bragg, S.P. Maheshvaranda, R. Nordemar, V. Preobrashenskiy "Spine – the Key to your Health", 1996, St.Petersburg

E.S. Velhover, G.V. Kushneer, "Skin - Mirror of Ilnesses", 1996, St.Petersburg

Yosiro Zuzumi, "Keeping Health by Finger Exercises", 1996, St.Petersburg

Jacke de Langr "A Practical Course of Do-In System", 1996, St.Petersburg

Tokuiro Namikoshi "Shiatsu. Japanese Therapy by Finger Pressure", 1996, St.Petersburg

F. M. Hauston "Healing with the Help of Acupressure", 1996, St.Petersburg

P.P. Sokolov, U. N. Gerasimov "Auricolotherapy, Or Micromassage of Ear Points", 1996, St.Petersburg

Pamela Jannett "Human Body", 2004, Huntington Beach, Creative Teaching Press Inc.